SECRETS OF A HEALTHY HEART.

9 effective techniques to fast & naturally enhance your heart health.

By

Kelly P. King

TABLE OF CONTENT

part 2
How to Maintain a Healthy Heart naturally

- the heart rate.

- degrees of cholesterol.

- test for type 2 diabetes.

INTRODUCTION

One of the main causes of death in America is heart attacks.

Given that the majority of us experience various types of health conditions

It is no surprise that many of us are merely ticking time bombs before we can suffer a heart attack ourselves since we are putting a lot of additional stress on the heart through our lack of exercise and unhealthy eating habits.

Your heart and the rest of your body were developed by Mother Nature over hundreds of thousands of years of evolution.

Nature has refined this organ to become possibly the most vital one in your body.
The heart is a powerful muscle that moves blood throughout the body, carrying oxygen and other nutrients to all the organs and cells.
Also, it offers a way to get rid of the waste that is created by daily body functions.

The numerous facets of heart disease and heart attacks will be briefly discussed in this manual.
You'll discover

all the information you require regarding heart attacks,
some of the difficulties that may result from them, and
even the risk factors that may increase your risk of
developing a heart attack.

At some time, attack.
But, the good news is that there are numerous things
you can do to lessen your risk of having a heart attack;
you just need to get started as soon as you can.
In this manual, we'll look at a few of the things you can
do to maintain heart health and quickly feel better.

Having a strong heart and living a long, healthy life are
goals shared by everyone.
When you are prepared to avoid heart attacks and feel
as good as possible, be sure to read this manual and
discover the actions you should take to start seeing
results and maintaining a healthy heart.

Chapter 1

WHAT IS A HEART ATTACK OR STROKE "MYOCARDIAL INFARCTION"

A heart attack happens when a section of the heart muscle dies or becomes necrotic as a result of the blood supply being cut off.
When a coronary artery, which supplies blood to the heart muscle through blood clots, is blocked, the blood supply is typically lost.
A different name for this ailment is coronary thrombosis.

When this occurs, unpleasant symptoms such as chest discomfort and electrical instability of the myocardial tissues are experienced.

Heart disease is a fairly broad phrase used to refer to all the various conditions and illnesses that can harm your heart and its function.
The blockage of the arteries that bring oxygen-rich blood from the lungs to the heart is one of the most frequent causes of oxygen starvation, which is one of the most common symptoms.
If neglected, this illness might cause damage to the heart, which can result in necrosis.
To put it another way, the cardiac cells will begin to die.

This illness can occasionally be brought on by the accumulation of plaque, a waxy substance.

Your arteries might become clogged with plaque, which can lead to the

partial or complete blockage of coronary (or heart) arteries.

Atherosclerosis is the name given to this condition.
Your organs and tissues' blood flow will be constrained as a result.
The parts of the heart that depend on this artery will die if this problem is not treated right away.
The once-healthy heart tissues will also experience fibrosis, resulting in scarring that impairs the heart's regular operations.

Such a problem can occasionally slip under the radar and be challenging to find.
Long-term heart health issues will therefore develop if you leave things as they are now.

Heart Attack or MI Symptoms:

Many individuals are searching for methods to prevent heart attacks because there are so many people who experience them.
But first, we should become familiar with the early indicators and symptoms of a heart attack or MI.

There are many different heart attack signs and symptoms.
For instance, although someone else may be experiencing agonizing discomfort, you may simply have minor chest pain.

Men and women alike frequently experience heaviness, soreness, pressure, and even discomfort in the chest, beneath the breastbone, or in the arm.

discomfort that spreads to the jaw, throat, arm, or back.

feeling bloated, full, and possibly even like I'm choking. Sometimes it could feel like heartburn.

Sweating, nausea, vomiting, and dizziness.

extreme breathlessness, nervousness, or weakness.

Lose consciousness or collapse.

How to Recognize a MI or Heart Attack?:

Each year, hundreds of people succumb to heart attacks without even being aware that they are experiencing one.

Since the majority of people who have had heart attacks in their early stages are asymptomatic until the crisis occurs, they behave as if nothing has happened.

Consider it a ticking time bomb.
We examine the signs and symptoms a person exhibits
to diagnose any disorders.
Each person has their own unique set of heart attack
symptoms.
They may be minor or serious.
Moreover, factors like age, sex, the presence of risk
factors, or underlying conditions affect how serious the
disease is and how susceptible a person is to get it.
For example, people with diabetes typically have subtle
or atypical symptoms.

In any event, you must seek emergency care right away
if you experience any heart attack symptoms.
The expediency of treatment is crucial when managing

attacks on the heart on occasion.
The likelihood of survival increases with the speed of
emergency care.

Remind yourself to ask for assistance from others if you
are experiencing an attack.
When you're in agonizing agony, don't try to drive or
walk yourself to the hospital because you'll just
aggravate the symptoms and invite further issues.
Ask someone to call an ambulance so you can get help
right away.
By getting immediate medical attention, you can stop
more damage to your heart tissues and perhaps prolong
your life because every second matters.

Cardiogenic vs. Non-cardiogenic Chest Pain:

Throughout their lives, the majority of people will, to some degree, experience chest pain.
Due to the frequent connection between chest pain and heart illness, worry frequently causes this.
Thankfully, practically all chest pain has little to do with the heart, but you should still pay attention to it.

The diagnosis of heart disorders is aided by an understanding of the variations in chest discomfort.
One of the initial indications that the disease is present is a pain in the left side of the chest.
Identifying whether the discomfort is caused by the heart or by other sources is the next stage.

There are several distinct structures in the chest and lung regions, all of which may cause discomfort.
The muscles and joints surrounding the most frequent location for pain or soreness are the

a chest.
While the lungs do not have any nerve connections that might cause pain, the lining or pleura surrounding the lungs can be connected with discomfort if it becomes inflamed or irritated.

Another location of your chest where you may have discomfort is the esophagus, which is the tube that connects your mouth to your stomach.

While refluxing, often known as heartburn, has nothing
to do with your heart, it may frequently cause discomfort
that mimics a heart condition.

Spasms in the esophagus are also non-cardiogenic and
may occur or be caused by them.

Mornings are often when people feel chest discomfort
that is cardiac or heart-related.
A burning or squeezing feeling is one of the symptoms,
along with a dull, confined pressure.
Most often, patients discover that their chest discomfort
originates in deeper portions of their chest rather than
the more visible areas.
It might be difficult to pinpoint the site of the discomfort,
however.

The pain may seem to come from everywhere, including
the back, neck, head, throat, and even the arms—often
the left upper arm.
People often say that "the pain came out of nowhere"
because they are unsure where the suffering originated.

An exerting activity like sweeping, excavating, or
carrying a large bag might cause chest discomfort.
A heart attack may also be brought on by an extreme
temperature while working or exercising.
It may also happen after consuming a large meal and
engaging in strenuous activity.
Some kinds of discomfort often continue as long as

When the action that started is terminated, the physical activity that you are performing continues but often decreases relatively rapidly.

Certain heart-related pains, like angina, may be made worse by laying down, but rising, sitting down, or even leaning towards the painful spot can assist to alleviate it.

You must get medical attention right away if you experience this kind of discomfort or pain.
The end of the day or just before is when other kinds of chest discomfort that are unrelated to the heart most often appear.
The pain is generally in a single, plainly identifiable region and often seems considerably sharper than normal.
Other than engaging in an uncommon activity, this kind of pain often strikes with little to no actual notice.

Eating meals that are greasy or heavy in carbohydrates may cause heartburn.
These kinds of discomfort often come and go swiftly; they may last just a few seconds or minutes, or they may last for many hours.
This sort of discomfort may often be reduced or eliminated with simple exercises, particularly breathing exercises.
Analgesics like aspirin and heat packs will often work effectively to relieve the pain.

The Actions Your Medical Professional Will Take:

A series of questions about your age, sex, dietary habits, and medical history will often be asked of you by your healthcare provider.
Your vital signs, including weight and blood pressure, will be taken.

The ratio of your body fat may be ascertained using pressure, temperature, and perhaps a test.

If you are a 25-year-old gymnast or martial arts student who has just begun lifting weights and taking a bodybuilding course, it is reasonable to presume that the source of your discomfort is a muscle.

It is safe to assume that your doctor will be looking for a heart-related cause for your pain if you happen to be a 56-year-old male who is a heavy smoker and drinker, does little physical work, works in a stressful environment, has high blood pressure, consumes mostly processed foods, and has a family history of heart disease.

This is so because each of these variables raises the likelihood of having a heart attack.

You'll likely be required to take several exams and

potential chest X-ray to identify your issue and choose the best course of action for you.

If you've established that the chest discomfort is being caused by a damaged heart, get immediate help as soon as you can.

You may even be able to stop heart attacks altogether with early recognition of the source of the issue.

You'll have the greatest chance of making a complete or adequate recovery in the shortest amount of time by receiving therapy as soon as feasible.

Chapter 2

Serious Heart Attack Complications and Heart Failure

Heart failure happens when your heart is unable to circulate enough blood throughout your body to fulfill all of your physiological requirements.
All of the body's organs and sections may get harmed by heart failure in various ways.
The neurological system, skin, lungs, kidneys, and skin all have the potential to be impacted.
Veins in the arms, hands, legs, feet, belly, and neck may also be impacted and often swell.
Breathing problems may also be brought on by heart failure, particularly if you're working out.

Heart Valvular Disorder:

When the heart's valves that regulate blood flow aren't functioning correctly, it results in this ailment.
Your blood will flow easily ahead thanks to the heart's valves.

is impervious to backflow.
Each individual's healthy heart functions in the same manner.

Four chambers make up the heart, and each chamber's egress is where the heart valves are located.

Your left and right atria are connected by the mitral and tricuspid valves, which allow blood to pass through and into the ventricles.
The valves will close when the chambers of your ventricles are full, preventing blood flow back to the atria as the ventricles contract.
Aortic and pulmonic valves must open as a result of the ventricles beginning to contract.
The left ventricle's blood flows into the aorta, then, after passing via the aortic valve, to the rest of the body.
it's blood

via the pulmonic valve exits the right ventricle and enters the pulmonary artery.

Once the ventricles start to relax after they have finished contracting, both

The valves are closed.
This stops any blood from returning.

For a lifetime, this process keeps happening.
Heart valve disease may be divided into two categories.

When one or more valves are constricted, hardened, thickened, or blocked, this condition is known as valve stenosis.
It may cause the cardiac pump to become insufficient, which will result in a shortage of blood in various body areas.

The four heart valves may all experience stenosis.

Valvular insufficiency is the other typical kind.
This occurs when a heart valve does not shut or seal
completely, allowing some blood to seep back into the
chamber or be pushed back in.
If this issue becomes worse, the heart has to work
harder to pump the body's required amount of blood.

Although some heart valve disorders are congenital,
others may not be discovered until later in infancy.
Over a person's lifespan, further forms may emerge.
While the exact reason is yet unclear, poor diets and
sedentary lifestyles are connected.
The pulmonic or aortic valves are often affected by this
kind of illness.

They sometimes may have malformed leaflets, the
wrong size, or improperly connected.

Bicuspid aortic valve disease, in which there are only
two rather than three leaflets, may sometimes be
present from birth.
The valves are unable to open or seal correctly or firmly
as a consequence.

When birth and early life-normal valves alter or develop
problems, acquired valve disease results.

Many factors might cause it, however, the primary ones
include infections or

disorders, such as rheumatic fever, which is brought on
by untreated bacterial infections like strep throat.
This kind of congenital illness often progresses fast to
cardiac valve inflammation if left untreated.
Endocarditis is a different condition that affects the heart
valves and develops when dangerous bacteria enter the
bloodstream and start attacking the heart valves.
Typically, it causes scarring as well as the development
of holes and growths.
The use of IV drugs, dental work, surgery, or serious
illnesses all often allow this bacteria to enter the blood
system.

Mitral valve prolapse is yet another typical ailment.
It is estimated that 1.5% of the general population is
affected by this illness.
As a result of this disorder, when the heart contracts, the
mitral valve leaflets slide back into the left atrium.
As a consequence, the heart's tissues will enlarge and
probably start to leak at the valves.
Unless there are underlying issues, this condition
usually doesn't get out of hand or need treatment.

Certain sexually transmitted illnesses, including syphilis,
are another item that may harm the heart valves.
In addition, a variety of medicines and high blood
pressure are known to exacerbate heart valve
abnormalities.

Heart Failure Shock:

Whenever the heart's pump motion fails to quickly pump enough oxygen-rich blood through the body, cardiogenic shock results.

relating to your body's organs.
Data indicate that if prompt medical attention is provided, roughly 50% of those who suffer from this illness will live.

Usually, a heart muscle injury results in this illness.
The majority of the time, it happens to those who are experiencing a serious heart attack.
Only around 7–8% of patients who suffer from a heart attack will also have a cardiogenic shock.
People often die from cardiogenic shock rather than a heart attack when they have a fatal attack.

As a result of this "shock," the body's blood pressure is dangerously low.
A hypovolemic shock is a different form of shock in which Blood loss,
 generally from trauma, prevents the heart from pumping adequate blood.

Vasoconstrictor Shock:

A sudden relaxation of the blood arteries, known as a vasodilatory shock, results in a drop in blood pressure

that prevents the blood from being pumped to the places that need it.
A bloodstream bacterial infection or a strong allergic response to a particular drug may be to blame for this. Regardless of the source, this indicates insufficient oxygen is reaching their important organs. This may also happen when the neurological system is harmed by "shock."

There is not much time left before the shortage of oxygen begins to cause damage that is often irreparable.
It is likely to result in irreversible organ damage or death if it is not treated right away.

Call an ambulance if you know or suspect someone is suffering from shock so they can get care right away.

- respiratory embolism:

A blockage in the pulmonary arteries in your lungs is known as a pulmonary embolism.
A pulmonary embolism often results from deep vein thrombosis, which happens when blood clots from the legs migrate to the lungs.

A pulmonary embolism may decrease or stop blood flow to the lungs, making it a potentially fatal disease.
The likelihood that this disease may lead to mortality is significantly decreased with timely and skilled treatment.

Taking the necessary precautions to avoid blood clots in your legs is one of the greatest strategies to prevent a pulmonary embolism.
If blood clots develop, get rid of them right away.

- Arrhythmias:

The word "arrhythmia" refers to a condition in which the rhythm of your heartbeat alters.
When your heart is weak, this may occur.

Whether the rhythm is erratically rhythmic, overly rapid, or both.

Sudden cardiac arrest, often known as SCA, is the abrupt cessation of a heartbeat as a result of an arrhythmia.
It may result in a person losing consciousness and dying if it is not treated right away.

- Syndrome of a Broken Heart:

This disorder is often exacerbated by mental strain and heartaches brought on by losing loved ones, ending relationships, and experiencing

Rejected, often anxious, etc.

Hence, it is known as Broken heart syndrome.
Chest aches and shortness of breath are the most typical symptoms of broken heart syndrome, however, arrhythmias or cardiogenic shock may also occur.

Other shattered heart syndrome symptoms often don't mirror those of a heart attack:

• The symptoms appear suddenly after intense physical or mental stress. • The electrocardiogram (ECG) findings, a test to monitor the heart's electrical activity, are often different from the symptoms.

Who has had a heart attack?
Those who have previously had a heart attack, for instance, will have a profound Q-wave on their ECG graph.

• The left ventricle or lower left chamber of the heart usually moves abnormally and there is a possibility of ballooning, but there are no signs of blocked coronary arteries when tested. • The recovery is typically swift, taking only a few days or weeks as opposed to a heart attack, which typically lasts a month or longer.

When a person gets older, their arteries often get harder and lose some of their flexibility.
While smoking is one of the biggest risk factors for this illness, the exact reason is yet unclear.

In addition to a bad diet or a diet high in preservatives, artificial flavors, and colorings, chemically generated medications are thought to be a contributing factor.

- Heart Valve Aneurysm:

A blood vessel's weakness leads to an aneurysm, which causes it to bulge and fill with blood.
They often take the shape of a heart.

attack.
These often happen in the aorta or close to the base of your septum.
Heart disease may arise from a restriction in the body's blood supply as a consequence of this.
Aneurysms eventually develop a scar tissue lining, which often prevents them from rupturing.

Ventricular aneurysms often develop slowly.
Tiredness, a lack of energy, and loss of stamina are frequent symptoms.
Certain ventricular aneurysms have the potential to develop blood clots, which may cause fatal consequences.
As the blood clots separate and spread throughout the bloodstream, death is often the result.

Although some aneurysms develop naturally, others are brought on by a heart attack.
Blood clots that have developed around them may prevent the blood vessels, a stroke, ventricular

aneurysm, or arrhythmia, all of which may cause limited mobility and tissue death in a limb.

Chapter 3

HOW CAN EMERGENCY TREATMENT BE PROVIDED DURING A HEART ATTACK?

Pre-heart attack symptoms often may not show themselves outwardly.

Up until the latter stages, this illness often exhibits no symptoms.
A person may experience pain or discomfort in his or her shoulders and chest, as well as fatigue, lack of energy, trouble breathing, and other symptoms of a heart attack in its early stages.

While symptoms may vary from person to person, a heart attack is characterized by 15 minutes of severe discomfort on the left side of the chest.
The symptoms of males and women vary.
Using women as an example, they typically do not encounter any

tiredness, disrupted sleep patterns, shortness of breath, indigestion, and anxiety problems are among the symptoms of chest discomfort that are often experienced.

Call 911 immediately if you believe you are having a heart attack.

away.
Time is of the essence; do not delay.
Delays in therapy may significantly lower a patient's chances of making a complete recovery.

Get help from a skilled operator by calling emergency services.

Heart Attack Warning Signs: The Six

The question then becomes: How can you tell whether someone is having a heart attack?
You may keep track of the following six heart attack warning indicators.

- Chest pain or discomfort is a first indicator of a heart attack.

The most typical sign of a heart attack in males is soreness in the chest.
A tlght, heavy, or scorching feeling is often what they feel.
Heartburn or indigestion may also be experienced as a result.
The center of the chest is where this feeling often starts, moving to other parts of the body afterward.
Most of the timo, this soreness will pass.

Some individuals just feel discomfort or a dull kind of
pain that may become extremely acute, while others will
only feel discomfort.

- Discomfort or pain in other body parts is a
  second heart attack warning sign.

Moreover, various areas of the body, including one or
both arms, the back, the stomach, and the jaw, might
experience heart attack symptoms.

also the neck.
Some individuals, particularly women, may feel pain or
discomfort in their jaws or backs during an assault.

- Breathlessness, a third heart attack warning
  indication

Breathing difficulties are a typical heart attack sign.
Shortness of breath is a common side effect of physical
activity and exercise, but if it occurs when you're resting,
it might be an indication of a heart attack.
It is brought on by fluid leakage into the lungs.
It may sometimes be an additional symptom for
extremely tired women.

- Nausea, sweating, or clamminess, Heart Attack
  Symptom No. 4

After suffering a heart attack, many individuals experience nausea, excessive perspiration, or clamminess, particularly women.
These symptoms may also be signs of the flu, but contact emergency services right once if they appear suddenly or if you have other heart attack symptoms.

- One's overall sense of great weariness or weakness is heart attack indicator number five.

Sometimes, general weakness or exhaustion will be the first symptom you hear from a heart attack patient.
While it may not seem like much, the majority of people who are at risk for heart attacks often experience this warning sign before the incident.
Yet, due to a large number of reasons for weakness and weariness, this symptom alone is insufficient to diagnose or predict a heart attack.
Lack of oxygen, insufficient sleep, bad dietary habits, anemia, arthritis, and other factors may all contribute to it.

- Collapse or falling, Heart Attack Symptom No. 6

Unlike other chest conditions where this seldom happens, a person having a heart attack often passes out or becomes unconscious.

happens.

Once again, if you see someone fall and lose consciousness, take them to a public space and contact an ambulance as soon as possible.

- Early Symptoms of a Heart Attack

Before they occur, heart attacks often provide some warning (except with Heartbreak attacks).
The heart muscle may get injured and this can often occur days or even months before an attack is about to strike.

A potential symptom of heart disease is high blood pressure.

Persistent heartburn may be a sign of a cardiac condition.

reduced cardiovascular health and breathlessness

abnormally high levels of LDL cholesterol

Before a heart attack, one may feel fatigued or ill.

According to several accounts, many individuals feel like they're about to die just before having a heart attack.
This is fairly frequent and can be related to depression, which is also a very strong sign of cardiac issues.

In particular, for those over the age of 55, abdominal discomfort and indigestion are typical symptoms of a heart attack.

It might be difficult to determine whether you are having a heart attack due to the symptoms being identical in many other ailments or diseases.
Thus, be careful to look out for any further symptoms.
It is simpler to identify a heart attack the more symptoms you discover.
To prevent and treat illness, regular checks with your doctor are advised.

- Before help arrives, what to do:

It is stressful to endure a heart attack.
While undergoing a heart attack, individuals often experience extreme terror.
Hence, make an effort to maintain your composure.

The "W" position, which is when your legs are bent so that your knees are up and your feet are flat on the ground, is the optimum recovery posture. This position is when your back is supported at a 75-degree angle.

The Venus position, which involves lying flat on your back with your feet raised over your heart, is another suggested posture.
Your diaphragm expands as a result, which facilitates breathing and

- enhances the flow of oxygen.

Any tightly fitting garments should be relaxed once the wearer is at ease to prevent any constriction.

The individual mustn't move about; the optimal posture is to lie or sit comfortably without putting strain on the lungs.

Someone may be carrying aspirin or nitroglycerin if they are anticipating a heart attack.
Typically, they will be aware of the necessary dosage. Encourage them to ingest a little.

When a person's heart stops beating, CPR must be started, but the person doing the CPR must be properly trained.

The best course of action if you don't know how to do CPR is to perform cardiac compressions.
The likelihood of survival is significantly boosted when CPR is started as soon as the heart stops beating.

- How to Respond to a Heart Attack While You're Alone Yourself:

Calling emergency services should be your first course of action. Be sure to provide your location, name, and a brief description of the issue.

You should only call friends or relatives or other people
after you have called emergency services.
Follow the instructions of the emergency service
provider as they are qualified to assist in times of need.

- till aid comes, provide instructions.

One thing you may still do that could save your life is if
you are alone and do not have a phone.
It has been argued that if this self-procedure is carried
out improperly, it might worsen the situation.
There is an alternative, however, if you're alone and
there isn't any support around.

In the same manner that a cat would cough to get rid of
a fur ball, take a very deep inhale before coughing
forcefully from the bottom of your chest.
An individual must breathe deeply every two seconds for
this to be successful.
Taking a big breath, coughing for a long time.
Up till your heart finds its natural rhythm and beats
regularly, this process must be continued.
Until assistance comes, it is better to keep saying this.

By doing this method, a lot of oxygen is delivered to
your lungs, and coughing causes the heart to beat faster
and maintain the blood flow.
Your heart's rhythm will return to normal as a result of
this pressure applied to it around every two seconds.

So long as you follow these steps, you ought to be able to wait for assistance in a stable state of health.

Chapter 4

RISK FACTORS FOR HEART DISORDERS "

One of the greatest methods to be sure that you won't

experiencing cardiac attacks or heart disease is to get familiar with some of the heart disease risk factors. Your family history and age are only two examples of risk variables over which you have no control. To avoid heart issues or a heart attack, however, there are a few elements completely within your control. For instance, you may alter your dietary habits, way of life, and mindset to lower your risk of a heart attack.
• Genealogy or ancestry

It may be more likely for you to acquire a condition comparable to heart disease if there is a family history of the illness.

Due to a mix of genetics and poor lifestyle choices, including

The risk of heart disease might rise even more if you smoke and consume unhealthy meals.
You can lessen your risk of acquiring any kind of heart disease if you take the essential precautions to care for your heart.

Some women have a higher risk of developing cardiac issues after menopause.
Since they are generating less estrogen at this period of their lives, this is the reason.
As a result, people must adjust their diet properly to lower their risk of heart disease.

- The Consequences of Obesity:

The worldwide health issue of obesity is becoming worse.
Obesity increases the risk of acquiring heart disease by four times.

Moreover, those having a history of high blood pressure in their family

or diabetes will be more vulnerable to heart disease.

Obesity is now understood to be an inflammatory illness; it is often considered to be a sign or symptom of further health issues a person may be experiencing.
Not only an eating disorder, as it was often believed to be.
Obesity is a significant risk factor
for heart disease and heart attacks, according to research.

- A bad diet, eating the wrong foods, and blocked heart vessels

- Strikes:

There is little question that a poor diet or one lacking in many essential nutrients is a major factor in the alarmingly high rates of heart disease that have emerged in recent years.

today's reality for many folks.

Processing and the synthetic technologies used to raise our food have taken a considerable amount of their natural deliciousness from them.
The four "poisons" in most of our diets are processed salt, highly refined carbohydrates, high fructose corn syrup, and refined vegetable oils.
Combining these causes heart disease by clogging the arteries and blood vessels in the heart, lungs, and body.

- Cigarettes:

Most people appear to be unaware that smoking is a significant risk factor for heart disease even though everyone is aware that it may harm your lungs. Indeed, around one in five persons who pass away

due to smoking, from a heart attack. The risk of developing heart disease is at least four times higher for smokers than for non-smokers. However, women who use birth control tablets face significantly greater dangers.

A heart attack might also increase your risk of exposure to secondhand smoke. Smoke from cigarettes depletes your blood's oxygen supply. As a consequence, your heart's ability to get oxygen from your lungs will be greatly compromised. Due to the compensatory mechanism, your body activates when oxygen is not available, it also results in elevated blood pressure and an accelerated heart rate. In addition to damaging blood vessels and artery inner walls, nicotine is also known to cause unintended blood clots.

- Alcoholism:

A tiny bit of alcohol might be good for our health.

The following are some examples of health advantages:

• Reduces the chance of having an ischemic stroke, which happens when the blood flow to your heart is reduced due to blocked or restricted coronary arteries.

• May lower your risk of diabetes

Yet, physicians would never advocate drinking alcohol for those with heart disease.
Since 90% of patients who are permitted to consume alcohol won't be able to control themselves, this is the reason!

Chronic drinkers, they wind up sucking down the whole bottle as opposed to just a bit.

Drinking more than the suggested quantity is harmful; you can only benefit from a tiny amount.

Thus, how can alcohol aid in the prevention of cardiac diseases?

Consuming a little alcohol may assist to lower bad cholesterol (LDL) levels while simultaneously raising levels of good cholesterol (HDL).
Moreover, it aids in preventing blood clotting, thins the blood, facilitates easier bleeding, and may help prevent a heart attack, but only when taken sparingly.

- Increased Cholesterol:

Despite years of claims to the contrary, cholesterol is now understood to be healthful and has no connection to heart disease.
It's true that

one of the primary materials the body creates.
As cholesterol is necessary for the body to operate, it is important.
Examples of organs formed of healthy cholesterol are the liver and brain.

Self-production of cholesterol is possible in our bodies. Yet when we ingest an excessive amount of LDL, or low-density lipoproteins, or "bad" cholesterol, we start to have problems.

LDL is overproduced when people consume too many omega-6 fatty acids, hydrogenated vegetable oils, and processed carbohydrates.

LDL aids in transporting cholesterol throughout our bodies to the locations where it is required. Overabundance may adhere to the surface when there is too much of it.

Thus, not enough oxygen-rich blood reaches your brain, heart, and other vital organs. Arterial walls of the arteries become irritated and clogged.

- Type 2 Diabetes

Due to their propensity for having high blood glucose levels, people with diabetes run the risk of long-term harm to their blood vessels as well as the nerves that regulate their heart's blood arteries.

Diabetics are approximately twice as likely to have heart failure than non-diabetics, and many of them may acquire heart disease at a young age.

Your risk factors will be significantly decreased if you treat your diabetes properly, as is the case with all cardiac illnesses.

- Physical exercise:

Being physically inactive or engaging in very little of it is a key contributor to heart disease and heart attacks. Because they cannot burn,

the extra calories, which cause the accumulation of fat tissues. The body needs to engage in a certain amount of movement each day to be flexible, healthy, and in good working order.
Obesity is a condition that develops when the body consumes more food or energy than it requires over a prolonged period. Obesity may result in several disorders. Exercise is essential for keeping the body in top shape and is a wonderful approach to improving heart health.

PART 2

HOW TO MAINTAIN A HEART-HEALTHY LIFESTYLE.

Finding a fountain of youth is like taking good care of
your heart.
Maintaining good heart health will result in a long and
healthy life.
The average person needs 7 to 8 hours of excellent
sleep every night to keep a healthy heart since this is
when the body repairs itself and the arteries that supply
the heart are at their healthiest.

Your artery walls may get damaged if your blood
pressure is too high, which will lead to the creation of
scar tissues and a loss of flexibility.

The flow of oxygen-rich blood to your heart and other
organs may be hampered as a result of this scenario.
The heart might get exhausted more quickly the harder
it has to work over time.
Thus, it's crucial to keep your blood pressure within
normal range.

Pay attention to your nutrition and stay as far away from
processed foods as you can.
Don't forget to work out as much as you can at the same
time.

Good quality clean fuel, or fresh, healthy organic food and a few processed foods, are what the human heart needs to function at its best.

To further enhance your general health, substitute soft drinks with healthy beverages like fruit juices or plain water.
Balance your personal and professional lives.
Increase the time you spend with your loved ones, family, and friends.
Your mental and physical health will benefit from this activity.
To keep your heart healthy, monitor your vital signs at routine checkups.

Chapter 5

ADOPT THESE LIFESTYLE ADJUSTMENTS TO PROTECT AND STRENGTHEN YOUR HEART.

Everyone must choose and commit to making healthy lifestyle adjustments at some point in their lives.
Often, individuals do so when they become aware that their bodies are beginning to fail them, when they are suffering from a fatal illness, or when they are grieving the loss of a loved one due to illness.
Often, it is at this time in their life that they make the decision that is best for them and their family.

Living a life that is vibrant, youthful, and full of vigor is always preferable to one that is ill and dependent on medical care all the time.
Our heart health is significantly influenced by our surroundings.
Thus, moving to a different location is the ideal choice if your current living situation is unhealthy for you, such as if you reside in an area that is very polluted and has subpar cleanliness and medical services.

- Nutrition: The Value of a Healthy Diet:

Our bodies and hearts combine to make an incredibly intricate biological living machine that is much more sophisticated than anything that man can invent.

But, it requires the proper fuel and lubricant, just like any machine, to be maintained.
The adage "Your body is your vehicle for this life's journey" has you wondering.
You ought to respect your body above everything else as a result.
If you had to choose between using cheap vegetable oil and trying to fill your new car's tank with cheap, soiled old petrol, which would you choose?

Why then would you harm your body in that manner when you can always purchase a new automobile but not a new body (well, maybe a new heart, but what a pain and price)?
It seems sensible to only provide your body with the greatest nutrition, right?
Of course, I meant that your dietary intake serves as fuel.
Just choose foods that will improve your health, not harm iDiet.

- The finest exercises for your heart:

So what kind of exercise is the finest and most successful for avoiding heart disease?
There is evidence from studies that vigorous exercise

Along with a little bit longer intervals of active recuperation, this combination is not only good for your heart but also helps you lose weight, control your blood sugar, and become fitter overall.

You only need to walk for three minutes at your regular pace, then sprint for one minute.
Simple, high-intensity exercises may help you burn more calories, improve vascular health, and improve the body's detoxification processes by repeatedly increasing and reducing your heart rate.

A total-body, low-impact activity like tennis, squash, swimming, rowing, Tae Kwon Do, or another martial art is a fantastic heart-healthy workout.
They are all related.

Give your body a decent workout by engaging a variety of muscles while avoiding overworking any one part of it and forcing your heart to work hard to supply them all.
You may develop your ideals as well.

By adding slow intervals, you may create a program that matches your current level of fitness.

Exercises for the core, such as pushups and squats, serve to build a strong foundation for your body.

Individuals who are active all day are often healthier than those who exercise for 30 to 60 minutes a day and then spend the rest of the day sitting down.
Keep in mind, nevertheless, that not all workouts are beneficial to the body.
For instance, long-distance jogging or running on hard surfaces is arguably the worst sort of exercise, even though it strengthens the heart.
It's because these endurance-type activities exhaust the body rapidly and put pressure on your joints over time, particularly if you don't wear comfortable shoes or run in good form.

It is also not a good idea to undertake any workout for which you have not warmed up or trained.
This can only lead to unintentional injury and may even precipitate a heart attack owing to an adrenaline rush.
Instead of switching to a workout program you may not love, stick with the one you already have and make it better by adding to it.

- Stress management:

The link between psychological variables and heart disease and potential heart attacks has been shown by a large body of research.
Your mood might be affected by hostility, rage, melancholy, anxiety, and social isolation.

risk of a heart attack.

Your chance of having a heart attack might go up by 50% due to financial and workplace stress.
It was discovered during the 9/11 terrorist attacks that persons who experienced significant levels of stress immediately following the incident had a doubled risk of getting high blood pressure and a tripled risk of developing heart disease over the next two years.
After significant earthquakes and other natural catastrophes, similar outcomes have been seen.

- the environment, clean air, and water:

Those who acquire heart disease and strokes (a stroke is similar to a heart attack) are significantly impacted by water and air pollution.

(A brain assault).

Since there is indoor air pollution, staying indoors too much may not be as safe as you believe.

A variety of different substances contribute to pollution, including fumes from home cleaners, wood stoves, fireplaces, secondhand smoke, cleaning product vapors, paint solvents, pesticides, insecticides, and carbon monoxide.

A cardiovascular patient may have increased heart rhythm, chest discomfort, and abnormalities that make it challenging to exercise if they are exposed to low amounts of CO (Cardio Monoxide).
Indoor

Furnaces, dryers, gas water heaters, space heaters, ranges, fireplaces, and wood stoves may all produce carbon monoxide (CO).

There is evidence that a number of regularly occurring minerals in water may worsen the signs of heart disease or perhaps cause it.
Heart disease is unquestionably linked to exposure to lead, arsenic, fluoride, and chlorine.

Chapter 6

GUIDELINES FOR A HEALTHY HEART.

For both the treatment and prevention of heart disease, several natural therapies include a range of herbs and vitamins.
the atherosclerosis.

An important contributing factor to heart disease is artery hardening.

Most Western countries are affected by this illness.
On the other hand, atherosclerosis is very uncommon in third-world nations owing to the different lifestyles, accessibility to traditional meals, and use of herbal medicines.
The health of the heart isn't compromised by the chemicals and poisons found in processed foods, which is the most essential benefit.

Ubiquinone, often known as coenzyme Q10, is a substance that aids in the energy conversion of meals by our cells.
In modern diets, this substance is often lacking.
Although our bodies naturally manufacture coenzyme Q10, as we age or have lower cholesterol levels, the quantity falls significantly.

This means that by including Coenzyme Q10 in your daily stack, you can make sure that your body receives a proper amount of nutrients to support your heart and maintain your cells healthy.

By taking these supplements, you may help control your blood pressure and enhance heart health if your diet is deficient in magnesium and potassium.
Salt has a lengthy history in human history, as you may or may not be aware.
It has been crucial to the advancement of public health politics throughout the years as well as the growth of human civilization.
Although being esteemed as an ingredient for thousands of years, salt is no longer as highly appreciated.

throughout the previous century.
It is now ranked among the most hazardous substances in the human body.

Yet, subsequent research has shown that even despite the quantity

Regardless of how salt consumption impacts heart health, it still plays a critical part in maintaining a healthy heart and good health.
Eating too little salt over time may damage your health and lead to several ailments.

Hence, for better health, we should limit our salt intake.

- What about the source of our salt?:

Minerals are abundant in unprocessed, natural sea salt
or rock salt.

- The finest salt source we have for supplying our
  meals with a wealth of minerals is sea salt:

Due to the scarcity of soil that is rich in nutrients, it is
difficult to locate even a trace of good minerals in our
food nowadays.
We may thus receive the essential elements from the
Earth's seas by including a range of sea salts in our
meals.

Yet not all salts are healthy for us.
In actuality, table salt, which is extracted from the salt
reserves under the earth, is highly processed and bad
for human health.
Table salt that has been refined lacks
is made mostly of natural minerals and often has
additives to prevent clumping.

All of the minerals' health advantages may only be
reaped by you if you consume them in

by selecting sea salt that is "worth its salt," meaning
entire, natural, and from the ocean.

And that's not even mentioning the fantastic flavor it can provide to your favorite recipes.

- Supplements like fish oil:

The quality of many supplements, including fish oil, is typically poor and they may even be hazardous.
The reason for this is that they oxidize as a result of the extraction method utilized.
Before making a purchase or using any supplements, it is necessary to check their quality.
A healthy, balanced diet often meets all of the body's nutritional requirements.

Only when your diet is inadequate or when certain medical circumstances force you to have an insufficiency or deficit will supplements become essential.
Dietary supplements generally are safe, and

There may be some danger involved with using some of them, however, some of them provide health advantages.
Several of them are also anti-nutrients, meaning they stop the body from absorbing nutrients.

Fish that has been fished in the ocean and plants that have been cultivated organically contain omega-3 fatty acids, which are vital nutrients.

They often occur in nature in a 50/50 ratio with other natural fats, such as omega-6 fats, which are great for heart health.

When animals are grown in feedlots or factory farms without access to natural foods or sunlight, they lack numerous vital nutrients, which are present in eggs, dairy products, and shellfish.
In addition to lacking omega-3 fats, they also have a high concentration of unhealthy fats.

It is thus strongly advised that you incorporate supplements in your diet to meet your daily nutritional demands if you are not eating free-range organic food.

- the significance of vitamins:

One of the most secure and essential nutrients for the human body, according to health professionals, is vitamin C.
With the aid of a

your body will experience a comparable result from walking as it would from a daily intake of vitamin C.
Walking is a low-intensity exercise that may activate the endothelin-1 protein, which causes tiny blood vessels to contract.
Research has shown that those who take a daily 500 mg time-release vitamin C dosage may reduce

endothelin-1 activity just as much as those who walk often.

One of the vitamins that are water-soluble is vitamin B9, often called folic acid.
It's one of the crucial vitamins you need to take every day to meet your nutritional requirements.
We can store vitamins in our liver.

Our body will draw the necessary quantity of vitamins from this store regularly.
The extra vitamins are then immediately removed from our body via the excretory system.

One of the most critical bodily processes, including everything from the creation of essential energy to the synthesis of red blood cells, is aided by vitamin B9.

In addition, vitamin B9 has other health advantages such as building a defense against cancer, stroke, heart disease, and birth defects.
Additional benefits include the development of muscle, the production of hemoglobin, and the avoidance of emotional and mental breakdowns.
Natural sources of vitamin B9 include lentils, broccoli, Brussels sprouts, asparagus, and broccoli.

- Foods and Enzymes:

Since they are organic, biological catalysts that initiates, promotes, and speeds up biochemical events, enzymes are essential for every cell in our body.

Viruses, bacteria, fungi, and their parasites' protein-based defenses are dismantled by metabolic enzymes in the blood.
They are purifiers that fight persistent inflammation and shield the body from most illnesses, including heart disease.
Although our body makes millions of enzymes every day, we still need a steady supply of new enzymes from fresh meals.

You obtain a good mix of enzymes and antioxidants as well as fiber when you eat a nutritious, wholesome diet that includes plenty of raw, fresh fruits and vegetables.

Antioxidants are chemicals that emit electrons and aid in keeping your cells healthy.
The oxidation of cholesterol is halted by antioxidants. Oxidized cholesterol is in reality the

the cause of death.

Although oxidation is a natural biological process, it may be fatal if there is an excessive amount of oxidized cholesterol.

Why is it the case?

It's because, in contrast to other oxidation products, our natural immune system often misinterprets oxidized cholesterol as germs.
As a result, your body will go to whatever lengths to get rid of oxidized cholesterol from your system, inflaming the artery walls in the process.
As a consequence, it may result in cardiac conditions such as atherosclerosis.

While there are numerous known antioxidants, vitamin E is one of the most well-known.
Many studies have shown the powerful antioxidant properties of vitamin E, which may both assist prevent and even heal free radical damage.

- Organic Foods vs. Industrial Farming

The phrase "Factory Farming" may be familiar to you.
The time is now.

The "non-traditional" method of farming that emphasizes keeping livestock in close quarters is referred to by this phrase.
They can accomplish this aim by using current technologies to speed up animal development, enhance production outputs, and lower the livestock mortality rate.

The consensus in contemporary society is that factory farming is the way of the future for agriculture, particularly among company owners and investors. Another notable invention was factory farming, which was hailed for its high productivity, cheap cost, and ability to address a variety of difficulties.
Nonetheless, many are opposed to it and argue that

Our health and the environment suffer more as a result of industrial farming than it does benefits.
Animal advocates also speak out against industrial farming's use of inhumane methods.

- What then is the reality?

Following years of careful observation and in-depth research in the agricultural industry, it is discovered that the majority of industrial farming uses subpar ingredients and dubious processing techniques.

On the other side, there is a method of farming called "Organic."
This phrase describes a method of growing and producing agricultural goods that is more natural and less hazardous.
For instance, current agricultural chemicals like GMOs (bioengineered genes), synthetic insecticides, sewage sludge-based fertilizers, and petroleum-based fertilizers cannot be used to cultivate organic crops.

Animal byproducts, antibiotics, or growth hormones are not permitted to be administered to organic cattle.
Livestock that is raised organically must have access to the outdoors and be fed organic feed.
Anything less cannot be referred to as "organic."

So, organic agricultural goods are healthier for us and less harmful to them.
Eating more organic food and less factory-farmed foods may improve health and increase the number of nutrients preserved.

- The true tale about detox

If the necessary raw ingredients are provided, our bodies are highly adept at detoxifying themselves. Those that consume a balanced, nutritious diet

and abstains from eating excessive amounts of processed foods (a little quantity is not recommended, but the body can manage it if not overloaded) and will experience increased energy and heart health.

Reflexology,
reflexology treatments
 and mindfulness

Anxiety and depression are two psychological risk factors that may undoubtedly have a significant impact on the heart.

Risk factors for heart disease may be affected and made more likely by stress.

in addition to obesity, inactivity, and high blood pressure (BP), particularly when these factors are present together.

According to the most recent clinical research, meditation may significantly lower your chance of developing heart disease, a stroke, and even passing away by around 50%.
When it comes to preventing or even curing cardiac illnesses, they discovered that deep breathing and intense relaxation might be more helpful than any new super medicines.

The end purpose of meditation is to discover "Balance" inside our bodies.
Meditation has been shown to balance out our biomarkers in the body, although this may seem abstract and difficult to understand for the majority of people in today's culture.
Neurotransmitters and hormones are other names for these biomarkers.

Hormonal shifts and a neurotransmitter imbalance are often to blame for tension or discomfort in any region of the body.
This condition may be effectively treated with meditation.

Several individuals benefited from this procedure to
control their biomarkers.

What makes meditation so effective?
The practice of mindfulness holds the key.

The ability to concentrate your consciousness on the
here and now and everything around you, both inside
and outside, is referred to as mindfulness.

Being in the present moment at all times is one of the
fundamentals of mindfulness.
being objectively present to your feelings, emotions, and
actions.
The key to being calm and present is to practice
non-judgment.

Mindfulness has many advantages.
According to studies, those who consistently practice
mindfulness are more likely to live longer, have better
hearts and immune systems, and are less likely to be
fat.

Reflexology is another alternative treatment for heart
health.

Those who choose non-invasive treatment will find this
technique appealing.

Reflexology may even be very calming and soothing for
certain individuals.

If you know how to perform these self-relaxing methods properly, you may use them on your hands and feet whenever you want to enjoy the advantages without having to go to a reflexology center.

By keeping the body and mind in a state of homeostasis, reflexology aids in maintaining the two in harmony so that the body may operate at its best.
Using pressure at a certain pressure

Reflexologists with the appropriate training can restore your body to its natural balance condition and repair any malfunctions at specific locations on it.

Every area of your body may be stimulated by applying pressure to certain pressure points, including the muscles, tissues, and even the cells.

In the hands and feet, these pressure sites are also referred to as reflexes.

The body's many pressure points have an impact on various bodily components.
The pressure placed on your feet's reflexes is where you may relax and energize your cardiac muscles while also indirectly stimulating your colon and pituitary gland.

- Healthy Foods for the Heart

Several foods have the potential to significantly improve heart health issues, mostly because they are particularly rich sources of the nutrients and chemicals that naturally occur in healthy hearts.

artery cleaning, inflammation removal, and immune system stimulation.

• Avocados have a lot of good fats, and frequent consumption of its ingredients may regulate and stabilize blood cholesterol levels as well as keep arteries free and prevent blood clots.

• It has been discovered that asparagus works very well to cleanse the blood, lowering blood pressure and slowing the formation of blood clots.
The vitamins B1, B2, C, E, and K are abundant in them.

Pomegranates support the generation of nitric oxide, which makes it possible for a person's blood to flow more freely through their blood vessels. They also feature a remarkable variety of antioxidants that aid to protect artery membranes.

• Turmeric helps maintain the arteries clean and lessens blood clots while also reducing inflammation and arterial hardening.

• Polyphenols and antioxidants found in persimmons help lower levels of bad cholesterol (LDL) and triglycerides.

They also aid in clearing the arteries and bringing blood pressure back to normal.

Spirulina includes important amino acids that are vital for the immune system to function better, normalize lipid levels, and helps to control blood fat levels.

• Cinnamon may help lower bad cholesterol levels and remove plaque from the arteries and blood vessels so that it won't build up there.

• Broccoli lowers blood pressure, helps to regulate cholesterol levels, and prevents calcium from building up in arteries.

• Most people's risk of getting heart disease is considered to be reduced by up to 40% by consuming cranberries.

Since they contain a lot of antioxidants, they aid to lower LDL levels and raise HDL.

• Catechins, which are found in great quantities in green tea, aid to eliminate artery blockages while also slowing the absorption of cholesterol.
Other benefits of green tea include improved metabolism and cardiovascular health.

Chapter 7

YOGA FOR HEART WELLNESS

Yoga may be practiced for a healthy heart even if you are not a huge lover of the gym.
It is ideal to practice yoga under a yoga teacher's direction.
Keep in mind that it is recommended to stay away from yoga positions that cause your heart to beat too quickly.
Although your heart will have to battle against gravity to pump blood to your lower body, avoid practicing inverted positions.
yoga poses to reduce risk factors for heart disease
How yoga may stop heart disease and fight it
Yoga may help reverse ischemic heart disease.
A study shows that yoga may lower the risk of heart disease.
Yoga tips for a healthy heart: dos and don'ts!

- 20 yoga positions to maintain your heart healthily

heart patients may do yoga

The following yoga asanas start easy before progressively becoming harder and requiring more energy and power.
When you get to the last ones, your body feels more at ease and renewed.

Tadasana (Mountain posture) (Mountain pose)

Vrikshasana (Tree posture) (Tree pose)

Utthita Hastapadasana (Extended Hands and Feet Pose)

Trikonasana (Triangle posture) (Triangle pose)

Virabhadrasana (Warrior posture) (Warrior pose)

Utkatasana (Chair position) (Chair pose)

Marjariasana (Cat posture) (Cat pose)

Svanasana Adho Mukha (Downward facing dog pose)

Bhujangasana (Cobra position) (Cobra pose)

Dhanurasana (Bow pose) (Bow pose)

Bandhasana Setu (Bridge pose)

Sarvangasana Salamba (Half Shoulder stand)

Matsyendrasana Ardha (Sitting Half Spinal Twist)

Paschimottanasana (Two-legged forward bend) (Two-legged forward bend)

Dandasana (Stick posture) (Stick pose)

the dolphin posture

Plank dolphin posture

Sphinx posture

Shavasana (Corpse posture) (Corpse pose)

Mudra Anjali

The positions that follow start easy and become harder
with time, requiring more strength and endurance.
The last poses help the body unwind and regenerate.

(1) Tadasana (Mountain pose)

The Mountain position increases flexibility and
strengthens the heart.

(2) postures, trikonasana (Tree pose)

The Tree Pose helps to balance and relax the mind.
Yoga position relaxation is beneficial because a quiet
mind promotes stable, healthy cardiac function.

(3) Utthita Hastapadasana . Utthita Hastapadasana,
also known as the Extended Hands and Feet Pose, calls
for more balance, concentration, and strength.

(4) trikonasana (Triangle pose)

A standing yoga stance that opens the heart and
encourages cardiovascular fitness.
While breathing deeply and regularly, the chest
expands.
It also improves endurance.

(5) warrior stance: Virabhadrasana (Warrior pose)

The Warrior position enhances physical balance and
boosts endurance.
Moreover, it relieves tension by relaxing the mind and
assisting in controlling the heart rate.

(6) Utkatasana, chair posture (Chair pose)

You might feel your heart and breathing rate rising while
doing this yoga pose.
It strengthens the body by making it hotter.

(7). Marjariasana cat posture (Cat pose)

After the Chair pose, this yoga position is a pleasant
reprieve since it enables the heart rate to relax and
return to being gentle and rhythmic.

(8) Adho Mukho Svanasana, the dog (Downward facing
dog pose)

While it soothes the body and energizes it, this yoga pose is employed as a resting position.

(9) Bhujangasana . Cobra Pose (Cobra pose)

Compared to the Sphinx pose, this yoga position stretches the chest more and calls for greater strength and endurance.

(10) Bow Pose, Dhanurasana (Bow pose)

The heart area is opened and strengthened by the bow stance.
The whole body is substantially stretched while being stimulated.

 (11) of the bridge: Setu Bandhasana (Bridge pose)

The Bridge stance, which is less taxing than the Bow pose, encourages deep breathing and opens and enhances blood flow to the chest area.

(12) Salamba Sarvangasana, (Half Shoulder stand)

The half-shoulder stance calms the parasympathetic nervous system and opens the chest.
It is a revitalizing and relaxing position.

(13) Ardha Matsyendrasana (Sitting Half Spinal Twist)

The sitting half spinal twist alternately expands either side of the chest while working the whole spine.

Paschimottanasana (Two-legged forward bend)
(Two-legged forward bend)

(14) Paschimottanasana 14. (Two-legged forward bend)

The sitting forward bend, which acts as a resting position, lowers the head to put it in line with the heart, which helps to slow breathing and the heart rate while enabling the body to rest.

(15) Stick Pose Dandasana (Stick pose)

In contrast to the preceding poses, this yoga position promotes proper posture, builds back strength, and simultaneously extends the shoulders and chest.

(16) Ardha Pincha Mayurasana, the dolphin pose

To prepare for more heart-opening postures, the Dolphin position assists by building stamina and strengthening the upper body, making it a bit more challenging than Downward Facing Dog Pose.

(17) Dolphin Plank Pose,
The dolphin's plank stance causes the heart to beat more rapidly.

(18). Sphinx posture Salamba Bhujangasana's sphinx pose

The chest may reopen in the Sphinx position.
It is a gentle backbend that elongates the shoulders and expands the lungs and chest.

(19) Shavasana. (Corpse pose)

Every yoga posture includes a counterpose called deep rest because it gives the body and breath the chance to make the minute changes required for the system's general wellness.

(20) Anjali Mudra.

The Anjali mudra relieves tension and anxiety while opening the heart and calming the brain.
Also, it better gets the body ready for meditation and pranayama.

Heart problems and disorders are becoming more common everywhere due to fast-paced lives, fatty diets, and reduced sleep cycles.

Yoga for cardiac conditions is a healthy, preferable alternative to using medicines.
Therefore go for the healthy, side-effect-free option for a longer, more robust life.

Yoga is a great exercise for heart health!

Yoga practice offers many health advantages and promotes the development of the body and mind, but it should not be used as a replacement for medical care. Under the guidance of a certified Sri Sri Yoga instructor, it is crucial to learn and practice yoga postures.
After speaking with a doctor and a Sri Yoga instructor, practice yoga postures if you have any medical conditions.
Visit a nearby Art of Living Center to find a Sri Sri Yoga program.

- yoga asanas position that you need to avoid:

1. Chakrasana position. (Wheel pose)

Chakrasana is a backbend pose that needs a lot of strength and a consistent breathing rhythm.
It should be avoided since it puts strain on your heart to pump blood more quickly.

2.Halasana. (Plough posture)

In the halasana posture, your heart must also pump blood downward against gravity and under pressure.

3. karnapidasana. (The ear-closing pose)

The karnapidasana posture is identical to halasana, but it involves more work since you have to lower your legs so that your knees are near to your ears.

4. sarvangasana. ,(Shoulderstand pose)

While you are standing on your shoulders and placing all of your weight on your upper body, you should avoid the Sarvangasana posture.
For blood circulation, the heart must struggle against the force of gravity.

5.Sirsasana. (Headstand pose)

- The inverted pose Sirsasana.
The head is on the ground, the body is supported by the arms, and the body is maintained upright.
When the legs are supported above the heart, the heart must work harder to pump blood to the lower body.

6. viparita karani (Basic inverted position)

You must lay on your back in the viparita position, lift your legs, gently elevate your hips, and hold them with your hands.
In this posture, like in all the others, your heart may work harder to pump blood to your lower body since your legs are elevated above your heart.

Chapter 8

KEEP YOUR WEIGHT IN CHECK.

The chance of developing heart disease rises with weight gain, particularly in the body's center.
High blood pressure, high cholesterol, and type 2 diabetes are disorders associated with excess weight that raise the risk of developing heart disease.

Whether a person is overweight or obese, the body mass index (BMI) utilizes their height and weight to make that determination.
Being overweight is defined as having a BMI of 25 or greater, and this condition is often accompanied by higher blood pressure, cholesterol levels, and risks for heart disease and stroke.

A great technique for determining how much belly fat you have is your waist circumference.
The risk of developing heart disease is increased if the waist measurement is more than:

For males, this equates to 40 inches (101.6 centimeters).

Women's size 35 is 88.9 cm.

Any reduction in body weight is advantageous.

Only a 3% to 5% weight loss will help lower blood sugar (glucose), and lower lipids, and cut the risk of type 2 diabetes.
Blood pressure and cholesterol levels may be reduced by losing even more weight.

Chapter 9

ATTEND ROUTINE HEALTH EXAMINATIONS.

The heart and blood arteries may be harmed by
excessive blood pressure and high cholesterol.
You won't likely be able to tell whether you have these
disorders without being tested for them, however.
You may learn your statistics and if you need to take
action via routine screening.

- the heart rate.

Often, routine blood pressure checks begin in infancy.
To check for high blood pressure, a risk factor for heart
disease and stroke, blood pressure should be taken at
least once every two years beginning at the age of 18.

You will probably undergo screening once a year if you
are between the ages of 18 and 39 and have risk factors
for high blood pressure.
An annual blood pressure check is also offered to
everyone over the age of 40.

- degrees of cholesterol.

People typically get their cholesterol checked every four
to six years at the absolute least.

A family history of early-onset heart disease or other risk factors may need earlier testing than the recommended age of 20 for cholesterol screening.

- test for type 2 diabetes.

Heart disease is at risk in people with diabetes.
Your doctor could advise early screening if you have diabetes risk factors, such as being overweight or having a family history of the disease.
If not, screening should start at age 45 and should be repeated every three years.

Your doctor can suggest medicine and lifestyle adjustments if you have a problem like high cholesterol, high blood pressure, or diabetes.
Be careful to follow a healthy lifestyle plan and take your medicines as directed by your doctor.

CONCLUSION

We appreciate your purchase of this manual. I really hope you enjoy reading this book and get a lot from it. Generally speaking, maintaining the general wellbeing of our bodies begins with

of our hearts. By taking care of your heart, you will also be taking care of the rest of your body. Your heart health and general welfare will ultimately be impacted by the dietary and lifestyle choices you make. Also, your family will be impacted.
If your diet is mostly made up of processed foods, you are poisoning your body with toxins and empty carbs. Also, you might anticipate having serious health problems if you have a sedentary lifestyle and are idle for the most of the day.

You'll eventually shorten your lifetime if you have problems at some point in your life.
But, if you lead a healthy lifestyle and make wise decisions,

You may expect to live a long, healthy life free of heart problems and many other chronic health concerns that afflict the majority of people if you take measures with your diet and are involved in physical activity. As a result, you'll be able to enjoy your senior years in a state of generally excellent health.

9 798391 148739